How to Get Great Abs Quick!

J.B. Alexander

Legal Notice

The author and publisher of this book and the accompanying materials have used their best efforts in preparing this book. The author and publisher make no representation or warranties with respect to the accuracy, applicability, fitness, or completeness of the contents of this book. The information contained in this book is strictly for educational purposes. Therefore, if you wish to apply ideas contained in this book, you are taking full responsibility for your actions.

The author and publisher disclaim any warranties (express or implied), merchantability, or fitness for any particular purpose. The author and publisher shall in no event be held liable to any party for any direct, indirect, punitive, special, incidental or other consequential damages arising directly or indirectly from any use of this material, which is provided "as is", and without warranties.

As always, the advice of a competent legal, tax, accounting or other professional should be sought. The author and publisher do not warrant the performance, effectiveness or applicability of any sites listed or linked to in this book. All links are for information purposes only and are not warranted for content, accuracy or any other implied or explicit purpose.

Table of Contents

Chapter 1 - What Are The Perfect Abs?

You have probably been heard about "six pack abs," and know it is a good thing to have, but may be unsure of what exactly a six pack is. If you think that getting a six pack involves just beer, think again. And beer is the last thing that you need when you are trying to get the perfect six pack abs.

A perfect six pack is when your abdominal muscles are so defined that they are clearly identified. Anyone who looks at your stomach will see that the muscles are well defined and will be able to pick them out. There are six of them, three on each side of your abdomen and each one should look pronounced. The perfect abs are sought after more so by men than women who seek to get well defined muscle tone.

This is not to say that women should not try to achieve the perfect abs. To the contrary, women tend to worry more about having a flat stomach than men. Women can still have a soft look to their body and not a bulky, muscular look when they achieve the perfect abs using the methods described in this book. Women should not be afraid that they will bulk up if they practice these techniques. Instead, women who look for the perfect abs and follow exercise and diet to achieve this will look slimmer, will find that their clothes fit better and will have more confidence when wearing clothes or going to the beach. Six pack abs are for both men and women.

In order to get the perfect abs, you have to exercise and eat the right foods. There are a few short cuts that you can take to enhance your muscles and they will be discussed in this book. These short cuts, however, are not a magic pill that can get you the six pack abs overnight. There is no magic pill that you can take that can help you gain the abs of your dreams in a week. You have to be committed towards working hard to achieve this goal. The reality is that getting the perfect abs is all about hard work and dedication. If you are willing to work hard to have the body of your dreams, then you will be able to achieve it.

So, now that you know what the perfect abs are all about, you probably want to know why anyone wants the perfect abs. They are desired mostly for cosmetic purposes. Those who want to look their best without a shirt or at the beach want the perfect abs.

Some celebrities pride themselves on achieving the perfect six pack. These include stars of the motion picture industry as well as those in the sports world. They pride themselves on getting the perfect abs because they know the hard work it takes to define these muscles.

While women often want to have less definition and, by nature, have more fat than men, most women still desire a flat stomach and abdominal area. The exercises for the perfect abs outlined in this book, as well as the diet that you need to eat to achieve the perfect abs will be for both men and women. While women may not want the same extreme definition , these techniques will do them good as they will achieve a flat stomach.

Not only are the perfect abs something to be proud of cosmetically. New medical studies indicate that those who carry excess weight around their middle have more of a risk for heart disease and stroke. This goes for both men and women. It is therefore desirable for both sexes to have flat abdomens and try to achieve the perfect abs and carry less weight around their middle sections.

If you think that you can get the perfect abs through sit ups and a crash diet, think again. Getting the perfect abs takes training - real training that will entail you sculpting your muscles to the way that you want them. If you are the type of person who sets out to do something and then eventually does it, you will have a much easier time achieving the perfect abs. If you are the type who gives up at the first sign of adversity, then you will have a difficult time. Look for hard work in order to achieve the perfect abs.

Now that you are aware of what the perfect abs are, what they can do for you and the fact that it will take hard work to get to the point where you can have the perfect six pack abs, then you can get started on your way towards achieving the perfect abs.

Chapter 2 - You Are What You Eat

The first thing that you need to do when you are trying to achieve the perfect abs or any type of muscle definition is to watch your diet. You need to bulk up on protein and cut out the carbohydrates if you want to attain the perfect abs. This does not mean that you have to lose a lot of weight, but it does mean that you have to lose belly fat, which will get seriously in the way of your perfect abs. If you are overweight, you should want to take the tips found in this book to get rid of the weight and work towards sculpting your body. You will not only look better, but will be doing your health a favor at the same time. The main thing is that you want to diet for muscle.

So how do you diet for muscle? You certainly do not want to starve yourself as this will not do anything to help muscle definition. You need to eat sensibly when you are seeking the perfect abs or any other type of body building. And make no mistake about it - you are body building when you are looking for a six pack. This is part of sculpting your body muscles so that they look attractive and are well defined.

Foods that are high in protein are good for bulking up muscle and also losing fat. These foods tend to trick the body into thinking that it is getting more fuel that it is actually receiving. You should embark on a high protein diet if you want to build up your abdominal muscles. You will notice that body builders and athletes drink raw eggs. While this may be disgusting to you, there is a lot of protein in those raw eggs that gives the athlete or body builder strength. The body builder will need this in order to bulk up. You need to remain strong if you are going to define your abdominal muscles so that you have a firm six pack.

Foods that are high in proteins consist of the following:

•Meats
•Fish
•Poultry
•Nuts
•Legumes
•Eggs

All of these are very high in protein and will help you not only get energy, but will also help you bulk up. You can also eat foods that are fortified with protein. This includes foods that do not normally contain protein but have protein added.

One of the best foods to teat when you are trying to bulk up and create six pack abs is fish. Especially fish that is high in Omega 3 oils such as the fatty fish. These are not only an excellent source of protein, but are also good for the heart and digestive tract. There is even evidence that fatty fish can help you keep your brain healthier.

If you eat meats, skip the sauces and the breads. Just eat the protein when you are on a high protein diet. This will give the body energy and get the metabolism to start burning fat. Only it won't be getting fat from carbohydrates and foods that are processed quickly and turn to fat. So the body will start burning the proteins. You will lose weight in your belly this way that will help you to define your abdominal muscles.

Eggs are also a good form of protein, although you have to watch how you cook them. Hard boiled eggs are low in calorie and high in protein and are a good way to get started when you are trying to attain the look of the perfect six pack.

People who are not meat eaters can eat legumes and nuts as a form of protein. It is a good idea to take protein in the morning to get your metabolism going.

Foods to stay away from

In addition to the foods that you should eat when you are trying to get six pack abs, there are also those that you need to stay away from. These include simple carbohydrates as well as complex carbohydrates. Dairy is also a product that is high in fat and should be limited. Take fiber by capsules instead of through breads or vegetables, as they tend to be high in sugars. You will want to eliminate all of the sugars from your diet when you are going for six pack abs.

Remember that it is important to eat all of the foods on the food pyramid. It is never a good idea to eliminate one type of food over another for a long period of time. When you are looking to build the perfect abs, you should concentrate on a high protein diet, but still eat vegetables as well as whole grains and dairy. But sweets have no place in your diet as they do not offer any nutritional value whatsoever. Simple carbohydrates are absorbed quickly and do not stick around long enough to give your body any sort of nutrition. Eliminate simple carbohydrates and starches from your diet if you want to have lean, rock hard perfect abs.

What to drink

In addition to watching what you eat, you also need to watch what you drink when you are seeking the perfect abs. Water is your best friend when you are trying to attain the perfect abs. Stay away from energy drinks that are loaded with caffeine, from so-called health drinks that are loaded with sugar and from alcohol. Many drinks that people consume contain sugar. This especially includes alcohol. Alcoholic drinks should be avoided when you are dieting to have the perfect abs. All alcoholic beverages have sugar in them and offer nothing by way of nutrition. Avoid alcohol when you are looking to sculpt your body and abdominal region.

If you take coffee or tea, eliminate the sugar and cream from the drink. If you cannot tolerate it in this manner, then skip the drink altogether and have water instead. You will find that whether you are looking for the perfect abs, or just looking to lose weight, water can be a great benefit. It will not only hydrate you, but it will also give you a boost of energy that you need when you are trying to sculpt your body.

How to eat

It is important that you eat more proteins in your diet in order to achieve the perfect abs, but when you eat is also very important as well as how you eat. You will want to consume most of your calories in the morning when you are eating to get the perfect abs. This is a good idea for anyone who wants to stay healthy as you will end up burning off calories that you consume during the day if you are active. You do not want to eat anything late at night as this is hard to digest and will end up staying in your system longer.

Chew your food very well before swallowing. This is not just something that you heard from your mother, but is something that helps you maintain a proper weight and also helps your digestive system. By properly chewing your food, you will find that you eat less and have fewer digestive problems.

Drink a glass of water before each meal. This will curb your appetite so that you eat less. Drinking water is good for you, as outlined above. When you drink a glass before each meal, you find that you eat less.

By beginning to eat and drink right, you are on your way towards building abdominal muscles that others will admire. Most of all, you are on your way towards not only looking healthy, but being healthy as well!

Chapter 3 - Crunches For Abs

Naturally, you will have to exercise if you want to tone your abdominal muscles. If you do not need to lose weight, you can use the toning exercises as outlined here in this book to help you get the sculpted abdominal muscles that you need. If you are overweight and want to lose weight to get the sculpted muscles, you still need to do toning exercises and will also want to work on some cardiovascular exercises that will be described later on in this book.

Crunches are the ideal way to tone your abs and are one of the many toning exercises that you should use on a daily basis to get the muscles in your abdomen taut. Crunches are the first exercise you want to incorporate into your daily routine so that you can have sexy abs.

If you are a woman who wants to have flat abs but does not want to have the defined muscles that you see on men, relax. Women can get sexy, washboard abs without looking like a man. Your abdominal area will be flat, but softer. And although the muscles will be defined, they will not be bulging like a man. Women and men both get different results from exercise routines. Using the tips and exercises here will get you the perfect abs, whether you are a man or a woman.

To do crunches, lay flat on your back and bring you knees up so that your feet are flat on the floor. You will then want to put your hands behind your head and pull up towards your knees, concentrating fully on the abdominal muscles. You should isolate the muscles as you are pulling up so that you feel the strain. You will want to do repetitions of 8 crunches. The first day, you might be only able to do two or three repetitions. Or you might only be able to do one. If it has been a while since you have worked out, it will be more difficult for you to use these muscles. But you will want strive to do as many reps as you can without hurting yourself. If you feel as though you are in pain, you should stop.

The purpose of the crunches is to build abdominal muscle. The way that you build muscle is to tear it a little, let it heal and then tear it again. This is where the pain comes in when you are doing crunches. You are actually building up the abdominal muscles so that you can have your six pack.

When you first start doing crunches, you will notice that it is quite a strain and that it is difficult. As you do this exercise every day, you will notice that it is easier to do and will start feeling the difference. You will not notice the strain any longer when you are exercising in this way.

The more you practice your crunches, the better toned your abs will become. Crunches will flatten and tone your abdominal muscles, but this is not the only exercise that you need to do in order to get the perfect abs. You also need to work on side to side crunches.

How to do side to side crunches

Side to side crunches will help to develop the sides of your abdominal muscles. Just as you move up straight, you will also want to move to the side. Start with one side and pull yourself up to lean towards that side. Do 8 reps, just as you would with the center crunches. After you are finished, work on the other side.

It is important, when doing toning exercises, to allow your

muscles to relax after each time you do your reps of crunches. You want to take a few deep breaths and relax the muscles after you are finished the toning. When you are performing the crunches, however, you want to tense up the muscles, effectively isolating them so that they will get toned.

Another way to perform crunches for perfect abs is to lean on one side and then lift yourself up, concentrating on the abdominal muscles. This will work the muscles on the sides. Remember that you want to work the entire abdominal area to achieve the look of a sculpted six pack. You need to do both front crunches as well as side crunches that are performed on your back as well as your side to achieve this look.

Crunches may seem difficult at first, but will soon become easier. You may want to increase your repetitions as you continue to work on your abs so that they will continue to be effective. The best aspect about using this type of toning exercise is that you will start to see the results of your efforts not long after you have worked on the abs. You can usually see a difference in your muscle tone after a week of performing these exercises.

Try to do these exercises every day. If you skip a day, for some reason, just pick up where you left off the next day. Do not get discouraged if you get out of the habit. It is more important to get back into the habit as soon as possible.

Chapter 4 - Leg Lifts For Abs

Crunches will work well to tone your abdominal muscles, but this is not the only exercise that you need when you are looking for the perfect six pack. In addition to the crunches, you will also want to use leg lifts to tone the abdominal muscles. Leg lifts can be done at the same time you do your crunches.

Lay flat on your back on the floor and put your hands to your side with your palms down on the floor. Lift both legs up as high as you can, even if it is less than an inch off of the ground. While you are doing this, you need to once again isolate the muscles in your abdomen and tighten them up.

It is always good to work in repetitions of 8 when you are performing toning exercises. The leg lifts will work well to tighten the muscles in your abdomen and define them. Like the crunches, you will notice the results from this type of exercise within a week.

After you have done the two leg lift, you can also do one leg lift at a time. This is often easier to do and will tighten the side abdominal muscles. Do one leg at a time and then the other, repeating the repetitions each time. As you continue to do leg lifts for abs, you will notice that the leg lifts get easier to do all of the time. You will be able to lift your legs higher and higher as you continue to practice this exercise.

As you continue working with leg lifts, you will not only notice a change in your abdominal muscles, but also your leg muscles as well. As you get better at this type of exercise, you can use leg weights on your ankles so that it will be more difficult for you to lift your legs. If you continue to use this toning exercise on a daily basis, you will notice that it becomes much easier to raise your legs each time. You can purchase leg weights at a sporting goods store.

Leg lifts and crunches are two of the toning exercises that you can use that will work towards tightening up your abs. These will work well in your effort to get the perfect abs, but must be used every day. It is important to concentrate on the muscles that you are toning while you are performing the exercises in order for them to work. By isolating the muscles and giving them total concentration, while working on this activity, you will find that the exercises not only get easier, but they start to produce results right away. You will be able to feel the results from the leg lifts for abs as your abdominal muscles tighten.

Chapter 5 - Levitating Lift For Abs

Another toning exercise that you can use to flatten your abs as well as define the muscles is the levitating lift. Again, you will be laying flat on your back on the floor with your hands at your sides, palms down. You want to lift both your legs and your head up a few inches, while concentrating on your abdominal muscles.

This is similar to the leg lifts and the first time that you attempt this exercise, you will most likely not be able to get much off of the ground. This can seem impossible at first, but as you continue working at it, you will be able to lift up your head and your legs at the same time. While this is similar to the leg lift exercise, it exercises another part of the abdominal muscles and will further work towards sculpting the abdominals.

When you are exercising on the floor, toning your muscles so that you can have the perfect abs, you should have an exercise mat. This is not only more sanitary to use, but is also more comfortable for your head and neck. You should try to do these toning exercises in repetitions of 8 each and work on as many as you can at a time. Do not get discouraged. Although these exercises may seem to be hard at first, in time they will get to be much easier. And you will get satisfaction by seeing toned and healthy looking abs!

If you are overweight and need to lose weight before you can even see your abdominal muscles, you should still work on these toning exercises. They will help tone your muscles and make it easier for you to lose weight. Toning exercises work well in combination with lower body cardiovascular exercises to give you the perfect abs.

Chapter 6 - Cardiovascular Exercises For Abs

In addition to toning exercises that isolate the muscles and give you the tone that you want in your abdominals, you also need to use cardiovascular exercises that will work on the lower half of your body, including your abs.

There are many cardiovascular exercises that you can use for the lower half of your body. If you are overweight and want to develop the perfect abs, the first thing that you need to do is to start to lose some of that excess weight. We have already talked about proper diet and nutrition, now we must talk about cardiovascular exercise.

Cardio exercises are those that get your heart pumping and will help you lose weight fast. Cardio exercises should be performed in the morning or as early as possible in the day so that you can get your metabolism going and also burn more calories during the day. You should never perform cardiovascular exercises right before bed as you will find it difficult to go to sleep. You should also never perform cardiovascular exercises after you have eaten or it can give you a cramp. If you cannot set your alarm early so that you can get up to work on cardio exercises, you should do them when you get home from work and before you eat. This will help you burn off calories and will also tone your lower body.

This is not to say that the cardio exercises that you do cannot work for your upper body, too. Some cardio machines will work both the lower and upper part of the body, while others will tone the lower half of the body. You want to make sure that whatever type of machine you use, you will be toning the lower half of your body.

You can purchase your own cardio machine or you can join a gym and give yourself the workout that you need to tone up your abs. Or you can join a gym and have access to several machines. You will find that the gym is comprised of many exercise machines that can help you get the abs that you want as well as help you lose weight.

Even if you are not overweight, you should still exercise using cardiovascular machines for your abs. This will give you an intense workout that will help sculpt your abs faster and easier. There are some gyms around that charge a low monthly fee for membership. Not only will you get access to the cardio machines that will help you burn calories as well as tone up your lower body half, but you can also get access to weight machines that we will talk about in the next chapter.

Some of the cardio exercise machines that you can use that will tone up your lower half and give you the abs that you want are the following:

•Stair stepping machine
•Elliptical machine
•Rowing Machine
•Treadmill
•Exercise Bike

All five of these cardiovascular machines will work to not only get you slimmer, but also to tone up your abdominal muscles. You can use some or all of them to get the abs that you want. Most people find a machine that they like and settle into a routine. You can do that to help you get your tummy flatter than ever and start to get that six pack that you have always wanted.

Stair Stepping Machine

The stair stepping machine was the exercise machine of choice in the 1980s and works very well as a cardiovascular machine as well as a lower body toner. You can get your abdominal muscles toned easily when you are using the stair stepper.

When you first start working on the stair stepper, you will find that it is difficult to stay on this machine for long. There are several types of machines. Some of them actually have a rolling set of stairs that you have to climb while others simulate the climbing motion. Most stair stepping machines today will tell you how many stairs you have climbed as well as how many calories you have lost.

The first time on the stair stepping machine you will find it hard to stay on for more than five minutes, especially if it has been a while since you exercised. If you feel lightheaded or dizzy when you are using the stair stepping machine, or feel short of breath, you need to stop the exercise right away. Stair stepping is a high impact cardiovascular exercise. You should always discuss any new exercise routine with your physician before starting.

After you have used the stair stepper more often, you will notice that you can stay on the stair stepper for a longer period of time. You do not need more than 20 minutes on the stair stepper each day to get the results that you need. You can adjust the tension of the stair stepper to make it more difficult to use the machine and increase the tension.

As you get better and better on the stair stepper, you can also attach leg weights to your ankles so that you can increase the tension when you are climbing the stairs. You can continue with this exercise routine as you work to sculpt your abs.

As you are using the stair stepper, you need to concentrate on your abdominal muscles. Your abs should be first and foremost when you are using this machine to get the perfect abs. Pull your abs in as you are using the stair stepper and keep them taut while you are using the stair stepper for the maximum benefit.

In addition to exercising your abs, you will also notice that you can get firmer legs, buttocks and thighs when you use the stair stepper in this way. If you like the stair stepper, you may decide to purchase one of these machines for home. You will find that the more you use the stair stepper, the better toned you will be and the more calories you will burn. It will also get easier to stay on the stair stepper for the full 20 minutes as you continue.

Elliptical Machine

The elliptical machine will not only get your abs in shape, but will also exercise the lower half of your body as well as your upper half. The elliptical machine performs the motions of cross country skiing. This is a machine that is low impact and is easy to use. It will allow you to move both your legs and your arms at the same time. It is one of the most effective ways to lose weight using a cardiovascular exercise machine and can do wonders when it comes to toning your abs.

The elliptical machine will be easier to use than the stair

stepper as it is not as high impact, but it do the job. You will start to notice the results right away, but will not feel as out of breath or as much impact when you are using this machine as opposed to the stair stepper.

Many people like using the elliptical machine because they can do so without the impact to their knees and back that other machines give. The elliptical machine also allows you to move your arms back and forth, promoting more calorie burning energy.

Again, when you are using the elliptical machine, suck in your gut and tighten your abdominal muscles. You will feel the machine start to work on all of the muscles in your body. When you concentrate on a certain set of muscles and tighten them as you are working out, you can then expect to get better results in that area.

If you like using the elliptical machine to tighten and tone your abs, not to mention to lose weight, you may enjoy owning this machine. This is a fun machine to use and will work well to tone all of your body and work towards giving you the rock hard abs that you want.

Rowing Machine

The rowing machine is one way that you can also get your abs tightened up. It will also work on your legs, buttocks and arms. This is a high impact machine and will require you to mimic the motions of rowing a boat. It is an excellent way to lose weight and will help you burn calories. It is best used for someone who is reasonably good health and not severely overweight.

Some of the new rowing machines that you can use will tell you how much you have rowed and even allow you to race against other rowers. You can also learn how many calories you have lost and your heart rate with this type of cardiovascular exercise machine. The rowing machine can be hard on the knees, which is why it is best for someone who is not obese and having trouble with their knees.

Suck in your gut as you are rowing and you will feel the tension pulling on your abdominal muscles. As you continue to row, you will note that it gets easier and easier each time that you use the machine. While you may find it difficult to continue rowing for a long time when you first start out, after you get the hang of this machine, you will find that it is easy to use and even entertaining. You may decide to get one for your home to keep your abs as well as your other muscles in shape.

Treadmill

The treadmill is one of the most popular of all cardiovascular exercise machines. It is used for walking as well as jogging and running. Anyone can use a treadmill. One of the best aspects about using the treadmill is that it can be used by anyone to tone up as well as lose weight.

You should start out by walking on the treadmill and sucking in your abdominal muscles as you are walking on the treadmill. Whenever you are exercising on the treadmill, you should concentrate on the muscles that you want to exercise and tone and then focus on them when you are working on the treadmill.

The treadmill will tell you how far you have walked as well as how many calories you have burned when you are walking. This will also tell you your heart rate. The treadmill can be used for running, although it is just as effective at toning up your abdominal muscles when used for walking.

The treadmills that you get today are much more advanced than those that were made many years ago. You may find that you like the treadmill so much that you decide to buy one for your home.

Exercise Bike

The exercise bike is one way that you can tighten your abdominal muscles and also lose weight while toning the lower half of your body. You can get an exercise bike that allows you to sit straight up and down, or one in which you recline and have your legs in the air. Both of these exercise bikes are useful for toning up your abdominal muscles.

The new exercise bikes that are on the market today, as well as in the gym, are able to tell you how far you have ridden as well as how many calories you have burned.

The new exercise bikes will allow you to race against other riders that are depicted on the LCD screen. This can give you an added incentive if you need some motivation to keep pushing on when you are exercising. This can make using this piece of cardiovascular exercise equipment easy and fun.

Whenever you are using cardiovascular exercise machines, you should make sure that you are in good health before attempting the routine. You should talk it over with your doctor and see if you are healthy enough for an exercise routine.

If you feel any pain, dizziness or lightheadedness, you should stop exercising. This is something that can be a danger signal.

Start out your cardiovascular exercising slowly so that you can gradually work your way up to the point that you can work with these machines to keep your body trim and healthy and also tone up your abdominal muscles.

Chapter 7 - Weight Machines For Abs

You will notice, when you go to your gym, that there are weight machines that are made to exercise the abdominal muscles. These will work in addition to the other exercises and routines that were discussed in this book previously to help you keep your abdominal muscles in shape as well as tone and define the muscles.

When you are using the weight machines for your abs, you should use them every other day. You do not want to bulk up your abdominal muscles, but merely want to tighten them so that they look toned and defined.

There are several weight machines at the gym that you can use to strengthen your abs and tone them up so that you can have the perfect six pack. Two machines that work well will cause you to twist and tighten your abs and also to mimic the sit up routine. Because you can adjust the weights and tension on these machines, you can expect good results if you use them every other day to tone up your muscles.

Before you use any type of weight machine at the gym, you should be instructed on how to use the machine. Most gyms will have people who will help you figure out how to use a machine. They will instruct you on the right way to use the exercise machine so that you do so the right way. Using a weight machine incorrectly can end up causing you to hurt yourself.

Talk to a gym counselor before you start using the machine. Ask them how you can use the machine that will tighten up your abdominal muscles. The counselor may even have other machines that can be used for the same purpose.

When you start using the weight machines, you will want to use the lowest tension level or weight when you start out. Do repetitions of the motion as instructed and try to do 3 reps of 8. This will most likely be easy for you to do when you are first starting out, especially if you are using the lowest weight or tension on the machine.

You may not think that the weight machine is doing any good, but chances are that you will feel tension in your abdominal muscles the day after you exercise. You will wait a day and then perform the same exercises again. You do not want to strain your muscles when you are using the weight machines for your abs or this can end up doing more harm than good. You just want to create a little tension.

After a week of using the weight machines for abs with success, you can then move up a level when it comes to weights. This may become a little bit more difficult, but you will want to use the same repetitions. Be sure to use both the twisting motion weight machines to exercise the side abdominal muscles as well as the front abdominal muscles when you are using the sit up machine.

Each week when you up your weight tension on the abdominal weight machines, you will notice a change in the abdominal muscles. You will start to notice a change in the tone right away as you continue on this path. If you belong to a gym, you will want to take advantage of all of the weights that they have available, including those that are used to tighten and tone abs.

Unless you have a home gym, it is unlikely that you will have these machines in your home. But they can be very beneficial when it comes to getting the six pack abs that you have always dreamed about. Just be sure to use them the right way so that you do not end up causing harm to your muscles and build them up.

By asking how to use the machines and using them in the right way, you can then begin to work on the abdominal machines to further sculpt your abdominal muscles.

Chapter 8 - Pilates For Abs

Pilates is a type of toning exercise that has been used by dancers for nearly 75 years. One way that you get involved in Pilates is to join a class. This is another way that your local gym can help you. Pilates are excellent when it comes to toning up muscle, especially the abs. If your gym offers a Pilates class, you can sign up for this class that can help you work on toning up your abs.

Pilates works well when it comes to teaching you how to isolate certain muscles and work on them to get them toned. More than likely, your Pilates class will not only work on the abs, but other muscles as well. Once you get the hang of the Pilates and how to use them, you can use this type of exercise routine to work on your abs when you are at home.

If you do not have a Pilates class at your local gym, you may be able to sign up for one at your local parks department. There are many people who are glad to teach Pilates so that others can learn this type of toning exercise. Pilates will let you concentrate on your muscles that you want toned and exercise them to the maximum of your ability.

Throughout this book, we have been talking about isolating muscles and concentrating on them when exercising, either with a cardiovascular machine, toning exercise or with a weight machine. You might be wondering how you can learn to do this. Pilates can teach you how to focus in on your muscles and make the most of your workout.

Pilates is a much more concentrated type of exercise than any other toning exercise routine. One reason why many people like to use Pilates as a way to sculpt their abdominal muscles is because they can get the same results from a 15 minute workout when using Pilates as they can get from a 45 minute traditional workout. Pilates are made to concentrate on muscles and tone them so that they are strong as well as sculpted.

If you are at a loss as to how you can learn Pilates exercises, do not have a gym where you can be taught or a class offered by the parks department, you can also learn about how to perform Pilates from watching a DVD. Rent a DVD at your local video store so that you can learn how to perform these exercises that can help you get the flat and very toned abs that you can show off at the beach.

Once you learn Pilates, chances are that you will use them in other exercise routines. Pilates are low impact and you will most likely not only appreciate the way that your abs look, but also the rest of your body if you use Pilates on a regular basis.

If you want to have the best looking abs, try Pilates. Many models and others who exhibit perfect abs swear by this exercise routine that will start to work right away. You will notice a big change in your body when you begin practicing Pilates and will not only exhibit perfect abs, but also perfect toned muscles in other parts of your body. If you want to achieve the perfect abs, you owe it to yourself to try Pilates - one of the best forms of exercise for toning muscles - especially abs.

Chapter 9 - Change your routine

As you are working on your abdominal muscles, you will notice that you reach a stalemate where it seems as if the abs are not getting any more defined. This often happens with dieters as well. Everyone who works on losing weight or trying to define their muscles will reach a point where they cannot get any further with their efforts, despite the fact that they are doing everything that they can do to achieve the results that they want. So what do you do when you are at a plateau and cannot lose any more weight or gain any improvement in your muscles?

The best way that you can avoid this problem is to change the way that you are doing things. Sometimes, your body gets used to a certain routine to the point where you cannot get it to perform an more. When this occurs, the only thing you can do is to change your workout routine.

If you have been using Pilates instead of machine weights, begin using them. Start changing the toning exercises as well and begin using another cardiovascular machine. This jolt may be just what your body needs in order to get back into shape. You need to make some changes.

If you find that you have reached a plateau when it comes to your quest for the perfect abs, you should use a different method of exercise to break up the routine. This will cause you different results. The same concept holds true for dieting. If you are on a diet and reach a plateau, you should change the routine that you are using to get different results. This works with exercise as it does with dieting. Do not continue on a plan that is not working. Look for a plan that is slightly different to further your quest for the best looking abs.

You should also watch your diet at this time. You may want to start eating smaller meals more often in an effort to get more energy into your body. This is one change that you can make that will help you attain the goals you have for yourself.

If you reach a stalemate when you are trying to attain the perfect abs, try something new. Try performing a different exercise, change your workout routine or change your diet so that you can once again start getting the results that you want.

Chapter 10 - Using Enhancement Supplements

Enhancement supplements are used by body builders, including those who want to have perfectly well formed abs, as a way to bulk up muscle growth. The way that natural enhancement supplements work is to increase blood flow to the muscles and allow you to get more from your workout. You can often get a more intense workout when you use enhancement supplements than if you just workout without these supplements.

Natural enhancement supplements are made with herbal ingredients that have been used for hundreds of years as a way to increase energy levels in the body. Anyone who is looking for a way to increase blood flow to muscles can use these natural enhancement supplements. You should not confuse natural enhancement supplements with steroids, a product that is created from synthetic hormones and should only be taken under the supervision of a doctor. Enhancement supplements are made from natural products whereas steroids that many body builders also take, are made from chemically created hormones.

Many people who workout and want to build muscle bulk enjoy using enhancement supplements as part of their workout routine. They can make it easier to work out harder for a longer period of time and give you better results from your workout routine.

Other people dislike the idea of using enhancement supplements because they do not give them the instant bulk or muscle growth that they expect. Many people who feel this way do so because they have confused natural enhancement supplements for working out with steroids.

Steroids are usually illegally obtained and should be avoided by anyone who wants to stay healthy. The side effects of taking steroids include increased aggression, organ damage and even mental instability. Men will notice their testicles shrinking from taking steroids and women will begin to grow hair on their face and chest. Steroids are an unnatural enhancement that many in the body building circuit use to get those large, unnatural looking muscles.

Six pack abs are not unnatural looking. They are a well defined muscle group in your abdominal region. You do not have to resort to any artificial means to achieve the perfect six pack when it comes to your abs. You can get these abs using the exercises and diet formulas demonstrated in this book without having to resort to any supplements.

If you want to feel as though you are helping your workout along, you can take natural supplements that contain herbal ingredients, no chemicals and are designed to allow for increased blood flow to the muscle areas. This will not do you any harm and may also give you a psychological boost as well. You can purchase natural enhancement supplements at health food store as well as some online outlets. Remember not to get anything other than a completely natural supplement and stay away from steroids.

There is no magic pill that you can take to get the perfect abs. They take hard work and dedication. If you are willing to put the time into exercising and working out for the perfect abs, and eat a proper diet that will also benefit you in this quest, you can have the perfect abs. But if you are looking for a way to get this look without any type of effort on your part, think again. No enhancement or magic pill is going to do it for you. Hard work and discipline will allow you to have the perfect abs of your dreams.

Chapter 11- Keeping Your Firm Abs

It stands to reason that once you have achieved the perfect abs that you will want to keep them. Once you get to the point where you are happy with the way that your abdominal muscles look, you want them to stay that way. You should continue to eat the right way, lead a healthy lifestyle and workout regularly. This is a good lifestyle choice for anyone - regardless of whether or not they have the perfect abs.

Many people who achieve this type of feat feel that they cannot ever stray from their routine without their perfect abs collapsing and turning to fat. While you will want to stay on your routine as much as possible and eat healthy foods, if you stray from your diet or fail to show up for the gym, do not panic. This does not mean that you will lose the perfect abs that you worked so hard to attain.

Keeping the perfect abs is more of a mind set than anything else. You will want to continue to diet and exercise and be mindful of the way that you look. Chances are, that if you achieved the perfect abs of your dreams, you have already demonstrated a remarkable amount of determination and ability to achieve a goal. You might even feel a little bit let down, now that the goal has been completed. Or you might think that you do not have to do anything to maintain this new body.

You should never feel let down because you have completed a goal. While the initial quest to achieve the goal can be very inspiring for many people, and get them all revved up to complete the goal, you can still have other goals that you can set your mind to that can give you this feeling. You should still stay within your exercise routine as you are working out so that you can continue to keep the firm abs.

If you feel that you can let your body go and abandon your exercise routine because you have gotten to where you want to get, think again. You will have a more difficult time getting back into shape if you let your perfect abs go to waste. Or shall we say waist? This is because muscle will turn to fat if not used. It is important that you continue exercising and maintaining your perfect abs that you have worked so hard to achieve.

It is not a good idea to fight hard to get the perfect abs for the summer so that you can look good in a bathing suit and then let yourself go during the cold months so that you can eat whatever you want and not exercise. This is not only not good for your body, but it will make things even more difficult for you when next summer, you once again want to attain the perfect abs. You need to maintain the perfect abs through the summer, through the fall and through the holiday season when you are eating and drinking things that you should avoid. While it is fine to indulge now and again, you do not want to break your routine to the point where you have to start all over again from scratch in achieving the perfect abs when you want to get in shape for swimsuit season.

Once you have achieved the perfect abs, you will feel good about yourself and will also want to stay that way. One way that you can do this is to take a picture of yourself with your perfect abs and how you feel. You can then post that picture on the refrigerator so that you are constantly reminded of how hard you worked to achieve what you have achieved, how good you feel that you have the abs that you have always wanted, and what you need to do, and not to do, to maintain the perfect abs.

Chapter 12 - The Psychological Factor

Achieving the perfect abs can do more for your brain than any other part of your body. Sure, your body will look good and you will be healthy looking as well. You will feel good about your health and happy about the way that you look in clothes. But the way that you feel mentally will be even better than the way that you feel physically. This is because you will have a renewed sense of self confidence. Not only because you are happy with the way that you look, but because you have set a goal for yourself and achieved that goal.

Few things enhance the confidence level more than setting a goal and completing a goal. This will make you feel like a worthwhile person and give you a higher sense of self esteem. If you want to feel good about yourself, one way to do so is to set a goal and follow through with that goal. The psychological impact of attaining the perfect abs will be enormous.

There is also a psychological component to achieving the perfect abs that you need to explore when you are trying to achieve this goal. How bad do you want it? You need to ask yourself how bad you want to have the perfect abs and what you are willing to go through to get them.

In order to achieve this goal, you need to want it very badly. Many people will complain that they cannot lose weight or cannot quit smoking. They are usually defeating themselves when they say this. Of course they can lose weight and quit smoking as this is done by people all of the time. If it was impossible to lose weight, quit smoking or attain the perfect abs, then no one would do it.   But people do this all the time. So it is not impossible unless you say that this is so.

While the psychological impact of achieving the perfect abs is very powerful, the psychological factor that enables you to achieve the perfect abs is very important in this goal. If you are geared up towards achieving the goal, believe that it is possible and behave accordingly, you will be able to have the perfect abs.

Knowing that you can do it and believing in yourself is just as important as eating right and exercising when you are trying to achieve this goal. The first thing that you will want to do is to recognize the goal for yourself. If you are overweight, find the right weight that you want to be and start to lose, based on the tips and secrets found in this book. Think of your perfect weight and make that your long term goal. You will have to reach the weight goal before you can attempt to define the abdominal muscles so that you have six pack abs. However, you can still continue with the same exercises and diet ideas described in this book.

After you have come up with the ultimate goal, you need to set little goals to get there. Each time you achieve a little goal, you will feel empowered and your self esteem will rise. This will make it easier to achieve the big, ultimate goal.

Instead of telling yourself that you want to lose 20 pounds, tell yourself that this is your ultimate goal, but your goal for the next week is to lose 2 pounds. Begin your regimen of diet and exercise and you will easily lose the 2 pounds. You will feel good about yourself as you have achieved a small goal that is on the way towards a larger goal.

The same way of thinking must be used when you are trying to achieve the perfect six pack abs. When you have reached your goal weight and are ready to define your abs so that you have the perfect six pack, start to break the goal down into smaller goals. It is often too overwhelming for someone to only focus on the large goal when they are trying to attain a big improvement in their life. And a perfectly sculpted body is a big improvement.

Instead of looking at the entire picture, break it down. Set your smaller goals so that you can achieve the large one by saying that your goal for this week is to make it to the gym every day and achieve a certain number of reps or maintain a certain amount of time on a machine. One of the best aspects about the cardiovascular exercise machines is that they can give you results right away as to how much time you have spent on them, the calories you have burned and the workout you achieved. If you try to attain a little bit more each time, you will be not only working towards your goals, but you will also feel good about yourself.

You will find that by exercising regularly and eating healthy foods you will start to develop a positive mindset as it is. Exercise is like a wonder drug and can rejuvenate you. You will notice that you have more energy and feel better about yourself when you are exercising your way towards the perfect six pack abs. Your entire body will feel and look healthier.

It may take a couple of months before you can achieve the six pack abs that you want, depending on your current weight and health. It may even take longer. But if you set small goals for yourself and work towards achieving those goals, you will continue to feel motivated about having the perfect six pack.

Occasionally, you might indulge in something that is not good for you or skip exercise. If this happens, do not let it deter you from your goal. One of the reasons why many people fail to achieve their goals is because they give up the first time they encounter adversity. They go off the wagon by eating something that they should not eat, or not exercising for a day or two and figure that they should just give up. People who diet and try to quit smoking also make this mistake. One of the biggest secrets to having the perfect abs is that you cannot give up. If you fall off the wagon, just jump back on it again. Do not beat yourself up over a failure because that is self defeating.

Hang a picture of the perfect six pack abs where you can see it every day so that you can continue to work towards your goal. Motivate yourself by small rewards for a job well done by giving yourself small gifts or treating yourself to something that you like each time you reach a goal. Have a motivation in mind for when you actually achieve the large goal, too, although having the perfect abs and achieving the goal of realizing this is reward enough for your endeavors.

Once you have taken the steps outlined in this book to achieve the perfect abs, you can use the same type of goal oriented motivation to achieve other areas of greatness in your life. As you see how you worked towards this goal, you will also see that it is possible to achieve other goals as well. Goals that, at one time, you might have deemed to be impossible.

Anything is possible if you have dreams, ambition and goals. If you are willing to do what it takes to move towards that big goal by accepting the challenges of smaller goals and overcoming them, then you have what it takes to do just about anything that you set your mind to in life. Including getting the perfectly sculptured body and gorgeous six pack abs!